# Bladder Infection Treatment

**A Guide to Understanding the Causes, Symptoms, Healing, and Preventing UTIs.**

**Mrs. Alice A. Lillibridge**

# Table of Contents

# Introduction

In a world pulsating with life's demands, there's an often overlooked but critical aspect of our health—a facet that quietly, yet significantly, impacts our well-being: our bladder health. Imagine a world where the pesky discomfort and challenges posed by urinary tract infections (UTIs) no longer hinder our vitality. Imagine being equipped with the knowledge and tools to navigate the intricate terrain of bladder health confidently. Welcome to a guide—a beacon illuminating the path toward understanding, healing, and preventing UTIs.

Dear Reader, nestled within these pages lies an empowering journey—a journey that seeks to unravel the mysteries surrounding bladder infections. Our quest begins with a robust truth: UTIs, while often dismissed as common nuisances, can substantially disrupt our lives. But fear not, for this guide is more than just a compendium of facts; it is a beacon of hope, a testament to empowerment.

Consider this your ticket to an illuminating exploration, a voyage through the labyrinthine world of UTIs. We'll traverse the landscape of causes and symptoms, unveiling the vulnerabilities lurking within the urinary tract. You'll discover the critical relevance of hormonal changes, hygiene practices, and anatomical intricacies, unraveling the tapestry of factors contributing to susceptibility.

But let me assure you—this journey isn't merely about understanding the problem; it's about actively engaging in its resolution. Our guide doesn't merely stop at the diagnosis; it extends a guiding hand toward healing and prevention. From antibiotics to natural remedies, from lifestyle adjustments to alternative therapies, this book encompasses a comprehensive arsenal—a treasure trove of strategies for combatting UTIs.

Picture yourself armed with knowledge—knowledge that fosters a proactive approach toward bladder health. And as we venture deeper into this exploration, we'll provide you with a roadmap—a blueprint guiding you through the chapters that unravel the intricacies of UTIs.

This guide isn't just informative; it's an invitation. An invitation to conquer fear, empower oneself, and embrace the proactive management of bladder health. Here, objections dissolve, and skepticism gives way to curiosity. The road ahead might seem daunting, but within these pages lies a treasure trove of wisdom—a compelling narrative that promises to enrich your understanding and elevate your approach to bladder health.

So, dear reader, prepare to embark on a journey—one that promises enlightenment, empowerment, and a future liberated from the shackles of urinary tract infections. This book isn't just a guide; it's a roadmap to vitality, a testament to proactive wellness.

Shall we embark together?

# Chapter 1

# Understanding Bladder Infections

Urinary tract infections (UTIs) are bacterial infections that affect various parts of the urinary system, including the bladder, kidneys, ureters, and urethra. Among these, bladder infections stand out as the most common type of UTI, causing discomfort and disrupting daily life.

Symptoms of UTIs serve as warning signals, alerting individuals to the presence of a potential infection. These symptoms may manifest as a persistent urge to urinate, accompanied by a burning sensation during urination. Additionally, individuals may notice they pass urine frequently in small amounts, often observing changes in urine appearance, such as cloudiness or a strong odor.

Swift action upon noticing these symptoms is crucial due to the risks associated with untreated UTIs. If left untreated, the infection might ascend from the bladder to the kidneys, leading to more severe complications. Therefore, seeking timely medical attention when experiencing symptoms of a bladder infection is highly advisable.

Health care professionals play a pivotal role in diagnosing and treating UTIs. Consulting a healthcare provider upon experiencing symptoms is essential. Early diagnosis allows for prompt treatment, which significantly reduces the likelihood of the infection spreading to the kidneys. Antibiotics are commonly prescribed as the primary line of treatment for UTIs. The choice of medication is determined by various factors, including individual health conditions and the specific bacteria causing the infection.

Commencing antibiotic treatment promptly not only alleviates the discomfort associated with UTIs but also helps prevent the infection from progressing to more severe stages. Typically, symptoms start to improve within a few days of starting antibiotic therapy. However, completing the full course of antibiotics as prescribed by the healthcare provider is crucial to ensure the complete eradication of the infection and reduce the risk of recurrence.

It's important to note that the duration of antibiotic treatment may vary based on the severity of the infection and individual health factors. In some cases, antibiotics might need to be taken for a week or more to ensure the infection is completely eradicated. Adherence to the prescribed treatment regimen is essential to prevent the development of antibiotic resistance and ensure effective resolution of the UTI.

## Personal Stories: Real-life experiences illustrating the impact of untreated UTIs

The impact of untreated Urinary Tract Infections (UTIs) can be far-reaching, leading to severe complications that significantly affect individuals' health and well-being. Real-life experiences vividly illustrate the consequences of neglecting UTI symptoms:

**Case 1:**

A woman in her 30s ignored the initial signs of a UTI, believing they would resolve without intervention. Over time, her symptoms worsened, but she continued to delay seeking medical attention. Eventually, the infection spread to her kidneys, culminating in a painful and severe kidney infection. She was admitted to the hospital, where she endured several days of intense treatment to combat the infection and restore kidney function.

**Case 2:**

A young girl experienced recurrent UTIs that weren't adequately addressed. Despite attempts at treatment, the infections persisted, and regrettably, proper measures weren't taken to tackle the root cause. Over time, the untreated UTIs progressed to a kidney infection, resulting in irreversible damage to her kidneys. This unfortunate consequence of prolonged neglect of UTIs has had a lasting impact on her health.

**Case 3:**

In her 60s, a woman dismissed her UTI symptoms, attributing them to the natural process of aging. Unfortunately, what she considered minor discomfort turned into a serious condition. The untreated UTI evolved into sepsis, a life-threatening complication characterized by the body's extreme response to an infection. She required immediate hospitalization for several weeks to stabilize her condition and undergo intensive treatment.

These personal stories serve as poignant reminders of the gravity of untreated UTIs. They underscore the importance of not underestimating or ignoring UTI symptoms. Seeking timely medical attention upon experiencing any signs of a UTI is imperative to prevent potentially life-altering complications.

The cases presented here demonstrate the diverse impact of UTIs across different age groups and underscore the urgency of addressing UTI symptoms promptly. Timely intervention is key to preventing infections from escalating into more severe conditions like kidney damage or sepsis.

# Chapter 2

# Urinary Tract Infection (UTI): Symptoms, Causes, Treatment

## In-depth Exploration of UTI Symptoms
### Urinary Symptoms:

*Increased Urinary Urgency*: A sudden, strong urge to urinate, even when the bladder isn't full, is a prominent symptom of UTIs.

*Pain or Burning Sensation*: Dysuria, a burning sensation or pain during urination, often accompanies UTIs.

*Frequent Urination*: Frequent trips to the bathroom with minimal urine output characterize UTIs.

*Cloudy or Foul-Smelling Urine*: Changes in urine color, clarity, or odor indicate the presence of infection.

*Hematuria*: The presence of blood in the urine can signal an underlying urinary tract infection or irritation.

Systemic Symptoms:

Fever and Chills: Severe or complicated UTIs can lead to systemic symptoms like fever and chills.

Back or Flank Pain: Pain in the lower back or side can indicate a UTI that has progressed to affect the kidneys.

## Differential Presentation in Special Populations

*Elderly Individuals:*

UTIs in the elderly may present with atypical symptoms like confusion, agitation, or behavioral changes rather than typical urinary symptoms.

*Children:*

Symptoms in children may vary and can include abdominal pain, increased irritability, or new-onset bedwetting.

*Immune-Compromised Individuals:*

Those with weakened immune systems may exhibit non-specific symptoms or systemic complications instead of classic urinary symptoms.

## Diagnostic Challenges and Considerations

*Overlap with Other Conditions:*

Symptoms of UTIs can overlap with other urinary conditions like interstitial cystitis, sexually transmitted infections, or kidney stones, leading to diagnostic challenges.

*Atypical Presentations:*

Atypical symptom presentations require careful evaluation and differential diagnosis to rule out other potential causes.

# Understanding Root Causes of UTIs
## Bacterial Causes

*Coli Infections:*

Escherichia coli (E. coli) bacteria, commonly found in the gastrointestinal tract, are the primary culprits behind most *UTIs.*

*Other Pathogens:*

Bacteria like Klebsiella, Proteus, and Enterococcus species can also cause UTIs, albeit less frequently.

# Chapter 3

# Bladder Infection - UTI in Adults.

Understanding the factors influencing the prevalence of UTIs in adults involves delving into the anatomy, physiology, hormonal changes, and comorbidities that contribute to their occurrence within this demographic.

**Anatomy and Physiology**

*Anatomical Differences between Genders*

In women, the shorter length of the urethra makes it easier for bacteria to enter and ascend to the bladder, increasing the susceptibility to UTIs. The proximity of the urethra to the anus also contributes to higher bacterial exposure in females.

Men, on the other hand, typically have a longer urethra, creating a greater distance for bacteria to travel to reach the bladder. However, structural abnormalities like an enlarged prostate can obstruct the normal urinary flow, leading to stagnant urine and increased UTI risk.

## Hormonal Changes

*Impact of Postmenopausal Hormonal Shifts*

Hormonal fluctuations in postmenopausal women can alter the vaginal pH, causing changes in the natural flora and making the environment more favorable for bacterial growth. This change in pH and a decrease in estrogen levels can elevate the vulnerability to UTIs in this demographic.

## Comorbidities

*Conditions Elevating UTI Risk in Adults*

*Diabetes:* High blood sugar levels can compromise the immune system, impairing the body's ability to fight off infections effectively. Diabetic individuals are at an increased risk of UTIs due to reduced immunity.

*Kidney Stones:* Stone formations in the urinary tract can act as a nidus for bacterial growth, increasing the likelihood of UTIs.

*Urinary Retention*: Conditions that inhibit complete bladder emptying, such as neurological disorders or anatomical abnormalities, may lead to residual urine in the bladder, fostering bacterial growth and UTIs.

*Weakened Immune Systems:* Various illnesses, like HIV/AIDS or immune-suppressing medications, can weaken the immune system's ability to combat infections, making individuals more susceptible to UTIs.

## Factors Contributing to UTIs in Adults

Several factors predispose adults to UTIs, ranging from lifestyle choices to medical conditions:

### Hygiene Practices

*Inadequate Cleansing*: Improper hygiene practices, especially inadequate cleansing after bowel movements or improper wiping techniques (back-to-front instead of front-to-back), can introduce fecal bacteria into the urethra and subsequently the urinary tract. This bacterial transfer increases the risk of UTIs, particularly in women due to the proximity of the anus to the urethra.

*Insufficient Post-Sexual Hygiene*: Not urinating or cleansing the genital area after sexual intercourse can allow bacteria from the genitals or surrounding areas to enter the urinary tract. This practice is particularly relevant for women as sexual activity can potentially push bacteria towards the urethra, facilitating their entry into the bladder.

### Sexual Activity

*Introducing Bacteria*: Sexual intercourse can introduce bacteria from the genital area into the urethra, leading to UTIs, especially in women due to the proximity of the urethra to the vagina and anus. This factor is particularly significant when partners do not practice good hygiene before sexual contact.

*Use of Spermicides or Diaphragms*: Spermicides and diaphragms, commonly used as contraceptives, may alter the vaginal flora, making the environment more conducive to bacterial growth. This alteration increases the susceptibility to UTIs in individuals using these methods.

## Medical Procedures

*Urinary Catheterization*: Insertion of urinary catheters, commonly utilized in healthcare settings, can introduce bacteria into the urinary tract, providing a direct pathway for infection. Prolonged catheterization increases the risk further by allowing bacteria to ascend into the bladder.

*Invasive Procedures Involving the Urinary Tract*: Certain medical interventions or surgeries involving the urinary tract, such as cystoscopy or urological surgeries, pose an increased risk of introducing bacteria into the urinary system. This risk is particularly significant if strict aseptic techniques are not followed during these procedures.

Understanding these factors contributing to UTIs in adults emphasizes the importance of adopting proper hygiene practices, promoting awareness of risk factors associated with sexual activity, and implementing stringent infection control measures during medical procedures. Addressing these factors through preventive measures, education, and adherence to hygiene protocols plays a pivotal role in reducing the incidence of UTIs among adults.

## Identifying UTI Symptoms in Adult

*Strong Urge to Urinate*: An intense and frequent urge to urinate, even when the bladder is not full, is a common symptom. This symptom often persists, causing discomfort or urgency.

*Burning Sensation during Urination*: A burning or painful sensation while urinating, medically termed dysuria, is a hallmark symptom of UTIs. This discomfort can range from mild irritation to severe pain.

*Frequent Urination with Small Amounts:* Adults experiencing UTIs may pass urine frequently in small volumes, feeling the urge to urinate persistently despite minimal output.

*Cloudy or Foul-smelling Urine:* The appearance and smell of urine might change, becoming cloudy, dark, or unusually strong-smelling due to the presence of bacteria or pus.

*Pelvic Pain*: Some individuals might experience discomfort or pressure in the lower abdomen or pelvic region, indicating inflammation or infection in the urinary tract.

**Systemic Symptoms (In Severe Cases):**

In severe or complicated UTI cases, adults may exhibit systemic symptoms such as fever, chills, or back pain. These symptoms often suggest the infection has spread to the kidneys or developed into a more severe condition.

## Atypical Symptoms of UTIs in Adults:

*Behavioral Changes in Older Adults*

In older adults or those with compromised immune systems, UTIs may present atypically with symptoms like confusion, agitation, delirium, or other behavioral changes instead of the typical urinary symptoms. This atypical presentation, known as "delirium without fever," is more common in the elderly and requires careful evaluation.

*Non-specific Symptoms in Immuno compromised Individuals:*

Individuals with weakened immune systems may present with nonspecific symptoms like fatigue, malaise, or general discomfort rather than classic urinary symptoms. Such presentations necessitate a high index of suspicion for UTIs, as they might be indicative of an underlying infection.


## Diagnostic Challenges in Identifying UTI Symptoms

*Overlap with Other Conditions:*

UTI symptoms can overlap with other urinary conditions or be mistaken for symptoms of other health issues, such as bladder inflammation (cystitis), kidney stones, or sexually transmitted infections. This overlap poses diagnostic challenges, necessitating a comprehensive evaluation by healthcare professionals.

*Atypical Presentations in Certain Populations:*

Certain populations, including the elderly or individuals with pre-existing conditions, may not present with typical symptoms, making diagnosis more challenging and requiring a thorough medical assessment.

*Importance of Professional Evaluation:*

The diagnostic process for UTIs involves physical examination, urinalysis, and possibly urine culture. Differentiating UTI symptoms from other conditions requires healthcare professionals' expertise to ensure accurate diagnosis and appropriate treatment.

Identifying UTI symptoms in adult populations requires a comprehensive understanding of both typical and atypical presentations. Timely recognition and professional evaluation are critical to differentiate UTIs from other conditions and ensure appropriate management, especially in cases of atypical or complicated presentations.

## Treatment Options Tailored for Adults

### Antibiotic Therapy

*Selection of Antibiotics:*

The choice of antibiotics for UTI treatment is based on factors such as the type of bacteria identified in the urine culture, antibiotic sensitivity, patient allergies, and medical history. Commonly prescribed antibiotics include trimethoprim-sulfamethoxazole, nitrofurantoin, fosfomycin, and fluoroquinolones like ciprofloxacin or levofloxacin.

*Duration and Dosage:*

The duration and dosage of antibiotic therapy vary depending on the severity of the infection, the patient's overall health, and whether it's an uncomplicated or complicated UTI. Typically, a course of antibiotics for an uncomplicated UTI lasts for three to seven days, while complicated cases may require longer treatment durations.

*Follow-Up and Reevaluation:*

It's crucial to follow up after antibiotic treatment to ensure resolution of the infection. Reevaluation may involve repeat urine cultures to confirm eradication of the bacteria and to prevent recurrent infections.

## Individualized Treatment Approaches

*Tailoring Treatment to Patient Factors:*

Consideration of individual patient factors such as age, gender, medical history, comorbidities, and any underlying conditions is essential in determining the most suitable treatment approach.

*Addressing Underlying Causes:*

Treating any underlying conditions that predispose individuals to UTIs, such as kidney stones, urinary retention, or anatomical abnormalities, is critical in preventing recurrent infections.

## Symptomatic Relief Measures

*Pain Management:*

Pain relief medications, such as phenazopyridine, can help alleviate the discomfort caused by urinary symptoms like burning or urgency. These medications provide symptomatic relief but do not treat the underlying infection.

*Increased Fluid Intake:*

Encouraging patients to drink plenty of water can help flush out bacteria from the urinary tract, dilute urine, and promote faster recovery. Adequate hydration supports urinary flow and helps eliminate bacteria more effectively.

## Prevention Strategies and Lifestyle Modifications

*Hygiene Practices:*

Educating individuals about proper hygiene practices, including wiping from front to back after using the toilet and urinating before and after sexual activity, can minimize bacterial entry into the urinary tract.

*Cranberry Products:*

Some evidence suggests that consuming cranberry products may help prevent recurrent UTIs by hindering bacterial adherence to the urinary tract. However, the effectiveness of cranberry products in preventing UTIs remains a subject of ongoing research.

## Alternative and Complementary Therapies

*Probiotics:*

Research indicates that certain probiotic strains may help maintain a healthy balance of gut and urinary tract bacteria, potentially reducing the risk of UTIs. However, further studies are needed to establish their efficacy.

*Herbal Remedies:*

Some herbal supplements like D-mannose, uva-ursi, and goldenseal are believed to have antimicrobial properties that may assist in preventing or treating UTIs. However, their effectiveness and safety require more robust scientific evidence.

## Complicated UTI Treatment Considerations

*Hospitalization and Intravenous Antibiotics:*

Severe or complicated UTIs may require hospitalization and intravenous antibiotics to manage systemic symptoms, such as fever or signs of kidney involvement.

*Special Populations:*

Treatment considerations for special populations like pregnant women or individuals with immune-compromising conditions involve additional caution and may require tailored treatment approaches to ensure both the patient's safety and effective resolution of the infection.

UTI treatment in adults involves a multifaceted approach encompassing antibiotic therapy, individualized treatment considerations, symptomatic relief measures, prevention strategies, and potential alternative therapies. Tailoring treatment to the patient's specific circumstances and addressing underlying causes are crucial for successful management and prevention of recurrent UTIs. Close monitoring, follow-up, and patient education are integral components of a comprehensive treatment plan aimed at ensuring optimal outcomes for adults suffering from UTIs.

# Chapter 4

# Urinary Tract Infections (for Teens)

*Anatomy and Vulnerability*

*Adolescents and UTIs:*

Adolescents, similar to adults, are susceptible to urinary tract infections (UTIs). Understanding the anatomical structure of the urinary tract is crucial in comprehending how infections occur. The urinary tract comprises the kidneys, ureters, bladder, and urethra, and bacteria can enter this system, leading to infection.

*Urethral Length and Vulnerability:*

Females have a shorter urethra than males, which poses a greater risk of bacterial entry into the bladder. This shorter length allows bacteria, primarily from the gastrointestinal tract or external environment, to ascend more easily into the bladder, increasing susceptibility to UTIs in adolescent females.

*Hormonal Changes and UTIs:*

Hormonal changes during puberty, particularly in females, can impact the urinary system. Fluctuations in hormones may affect the pH balance of the genital area and urinary tract, potentially making it more hospitable for bacterial growth and increasing the risk of UTIs.

*Sexual Activity and UTI Risk:*

Engaging in sexual activity can introduce bacteria into the urinary tract, leading to a higher risk of UTIs in sexually active adolescents. Inadequate hygiene practices or irritation caused by certain contraceptives may further increase susceptibility to infections.

*Hygiene Practices:*

Personal hygiene practices, such as improper wiping techniques (particularly in females, wiping from back to front), using harsh or scented products in the genital area, or infrequent changing of undergarments, can contribute to bacterial entry and UTI risk.

## Common Symptoms and Recognition

*Educating About Symptoms:*

Educating adolescents about common symptoms associated with UTIs is crucial for early recognition and prompt treatment. Symptoms like frequent or urgent urination, pain or burning sensation during urination, cloudy or foul-smelling urine, and discomfort or pain in the lower abdomen or pelvic area should be recognized.

*Awareness and Self-Recognition:*

By understanding these symptoms, adolescents can self-identify potential UTIs and seek timely medical assistance. Encouraging open communication with parents or guardians and seeking medical attention promptly upon recognizing these symptoms can aid in early diagnosis and treatment, preventing complications.

Understanding the urinary tract's anatomy, vulnerability factors such as urethral length, hormonal changes, sexual activity, and hygiene practices are essential in comprehending why adolescents are susceptible to UTIs. Educating teens about common symptoms enables them to recognize UTIs early, facilitating timely intervention and promoting better urinary tract health.

# Chapter 5

## Home Remedies for Urinary Tract Infections (UTIs)

UTIs, while often treated with antibiotics, also respond to various natural remedies that can alleviate symptoms and reduce the likelihood of future infections. Let's explore these home remedies that offer a holistic approach to managing UTIs:

### Stay Hydrated:

One of the fundamental steps in UTI management is ensuring adequate hydration. Drinking plenty of fluids, especially water, aids in flushing out bacteria from the urinary tract. The recommended intake is approximately 8 cups (64 ounces) of water per day. Adequate hydration supports the body's natural mechanisms for cleansing the urinary system, thereby reducing the risk of infections.

### Cranberry Juice:

Widely recognized as a popular home remedy, cranberry juice contains compounds that hinder bacteria from adhering to the urinary tract walls. Regular consumption of cranberry juice may contribute to preventing the recurrence of UTIs. The active components in cranberries, such as proanthocyanidins, are believed to interfere with the attachment of bacteria, potentially reducing the risk of infection.

## Probiotics:

These beneficial bacteria play a crucial role in maintaining a healthy balance of microorganisms in the body, including the urinary tract. Probiotics can aid in bolstering the body's natural defense mechanisms against UTIs. Consuming probiotic supplements or incorporating probiotic-rich foods into your diet, such as yogurt, kefir, or fermented foods, may help in promoting the growth of beneficial bacteria, thus potentially reducing the risk of UTIs.

## Vitamin C:

This essential vitamin plays a pivotal role in maintaining overall health and boosting the immune system. Specifically concerning UTIs, vitamin C helps in making urine more acidic. A lower pH level in the urine creates an environment less conducive to bacterial growth, potentially inhibiting the proliferation of harmful bacteria in the urinary tract. Incorporating vitamin C supplements into your daily routine or consuming foods rich in this nutrient, such as citrus fruits like oranges, lemons, and kiwis, can aid in preventing UTIs by creating a less favorable environment for bacterial growth.

## Garlic:

Renowned for its various health benefits, garlic possesses natural antimicrobial properties that have been shown to combat bacteria. Allicin, the active compound in garlic responsible for its medicinal properties, exhibits antibacterial effects. Regular consumption of garlic, either raw or cooked, may contribute to preventing UTIs by assisting the body in fighting off bacteria that could potentially cause urinary tract infections.

## D-Mannose

This naturally occurring sugar is believed to prevent bacteria, particularly E. coli, from adhering to the walls of the urinary tract. E. coli is a common culprit in UTIs. D-mannose works by binding to the bacteria, preventing them from attaching to the urinary tract walls and facilitating their elimination during urination. Taking D-mannose supplements can be an effective preventive measure against recurring UTIs.

## Hygiene Practices

Maintaining good hygiene habits is crucial in preventing UTIs. Proper hygiene, especially after using the bathroom, plays a significant role in reducing the risk of bacterial contamination. Wiping from front to back after urination or bowel movements helps prevent the transfer of bacteria from the rectal area to the urinary tract, reducing the chances of UTIs. Additionally, avoiding the use of scented or harsh products in the genital area can help maintain a healthy balance of bacteria and prevent irritation that may contribute to UTIs.

These home remedies offer natural, complementary approaches to prevent UTIs by either creating an unfavorable environment for bacterial growth, harnessing natural antimicrobial properties, or preventing bacterial adhesion to the urinary tract walls. While incorporating these remedies into your routine may aid in UTI prevention, it's essential to consult with a healthcare professional for personalized advice, especially if you have underlying health conditions or recurrent UTIs

## Herbal Treatments and Their Efficacy

### Specific herbs and their beneficial properties in treating UTIs.

Herbs have been used for centuries to treat various ailments, including UTIs. Here are some herbs that have been shown to be effective in treating UTIs:

### Uva Ursi

This shrub, indigenous to North America and Europe, has been utilized for centuries in traditional medicine to address urinary tract issues, including UTIs. Uva ursi contains compounds like arbutin and hydroquinone, which exhibit antibacterial properties and work to reduce inflammation in the urinary tract. These components are metabolized into a compound called hydroquinone, which is known for its antimicrobial action against certain bacteria commonly involved in UTIs. However, it's critical to highlight that uva ursi can be toxic in high doses and should be used cautiously and under the guidance of a healthcare professional.

## Cranberry

Renowned for its preventive effects against UTIs, cranberry contains compounds known as proanthocyanidins, which interfere with the adhesion of bacteria to the urinary tract walls. By preventing bacterial attachment, cranberry may reduce the risk of recurrent UTIs. Incorporating cranberry juice or supplements into your routine might assist in preventing the recurrence of UTIs, but it's essential to note that cranberry juice often contains added sugars, so opting for unsweetened versions is advisable.

## Goldenseal

This herb contains berberine, a compound with established antimicrobial properties. Berberine has been studied for its ability to combat bacteria, including those implicated in UTIs. Goldenseal can be consumed as a supplement or used topically to address UTIs. However, caution should be exercised with goldenseal as it can interact with certain medications and might not be suitable for everyone. Consulting a healthcare professional before using goldenseal is crucial to ensure its safety and effectiveness for individual use.

## D-Mannose

This natural sugar, structurally similar to glucose, is believed to hinder bacteria, primarily E. coli, from adhering to the walls of the urinary tract. E. coli is a common cause of UTIs. D-Mannose works by binding to the bacteria, preventing their attachment to the urinary tract walls, and facilitating their elimination during urination. Many individuals use D-mannose supplements as a preventive measure against recurring UTIs due to its potential efficacy in hindering bacterial adhesion.

## Garlic

Known for its potent antimicrobial properties, garlic contains allicin, a compound with demonstrated antibacterial effects. Regular consumption of garlic, whether raw or cooked, may assist the body in fighting off bacteria that could potentially cause urinary tract infections. Its natural properties make it a popular choice among individuals seeking alternative methods to prevent UTIs.

## Echinacea

Widely recognized for its immune-boosting properties, echinacea has also shown potential antimicrobial effects. While it is commonly used to support the immune system, studies suggest that it may have some efficacy in treating UTIs. However, echinacea can interact with certain medications, and its usage should be supervised by a healthcare professional to ensure safety and effectiveness, especially for individuals with existing health conditions or taking medications.

## Horsetail

Historically used to address various ailments, including UTIs, horsetail contains compounds with diuretic properties that promote increased urine production. The increased urinary output may aid in flushing bacteria out of the urinary tract. However, horsetail can be toxic in large doses, and its usage should be supervised by a healthcare professional due to potential health risks.

## Nettle

Similarly, nettle has been used in traditional medicine to treat different health issues, including UTIs. It possesses compounds with diuretic properties that promote increased urine flow, potentially assisting in flushing bacteria out of the urinary tract. However, like echinacea and horsetail, nettle can interact with certain medications and should be used under the guidance of a healthcare professional to ensure its safety and effectiveness.

# Chapter 6

# Bladder Infection - Kidney and Urinary Tract Disorders

Let's delve into an extensive exploration of the relationship between urinary tract infections (UTIs) and related disorders, specifically focusing on bladder infections, kidney issues, and other urinary tract disorders:

## UTIs and Bladder Infections

*UTIs and Cystitis*

*Understanding Cystitis:*

Cystitis refers to inflammation in the bladder walls, primarily caused by a bacterial infection. This condition is a prevalent manifestation of a UTI, where bacteria, typically Escherichia coli (E. coli) originating from the gastrointestinal tract, invade the bladder through the urethra. The urethra's close proximity to the bladder facilitates bacterial ascent, leading to infection and subsequent inflammation.

*Pathophysiology of UTI-Caused Cystitis:*

Bacteria, upon reaching the bladder, adhere to the bladder's epithelial lining and multiply, triggering an immune response. This immune reaction leads to inflammation, causing the classic symptoms of cystitis, such as urinary urgency, frequency, burning during urination, and sometimes hematuria (blood in urine).

*Untreated or Recurrent UTIs Leading to Chronic Cystitis:*

If UTIs remain untreated or if there are frequent recurrent infections, the persistent presence of bacteria and inflammation can result in chronic cystitis. Chronic cystitis involves recurrent or persistent episodes of bladder inflammation and can lead to long-term bladder wall damage.

## Chronic Bladder Infections

*Impact of Repeated or Untreated UTIs:*

Repeated or untreated UTIs can lead to chronic bladder infections characterized by persistent inflammation and recurrent episodes of cystitis. The continual cycle of bacterial invasion and inflammatory response damages the bladder wall, compromising its integrity and leading to chronic bladder issues.

*Consequences of Chronic Bladder Infections:*

Chronic bladder infections can significantly impact an individual's health and quality of life. The persistent inflammation and damage to the bladder wall may impair its ability to function properly. This compromised function can result in increased susceptibility to further infections, persistent urinary symptoms (such as urgency, frequency, and discomfort), and even complications like urinary retention or incomplete emptying of the bladder.

*Clinical Implications and Management:*

Managing chronic bladder infections involves a multidimensional approach, including antibiotic therapy to eradicate the infection, lifestyle modifications to reduce the risk of recurrence (such as improved hygiene practices and increased fluid intake), and sometimes prophylactic antibiotics to prevent further infections in susceptible individuals. Additionally, patients may require regular monitoring and follow-up to assess the effectiveness of treatment and prevent complications.

Understanding the progression from a standard UTI to cystitis and chronic bladder infections highlights the importance of early detection, prompt treatment, and comprehensive management to prevent the development of chronic urinary issues and associated complications.

## UTIs and Kidney Complications

*Pyelonephritis:*

*Understanding Pyelonephritis:*

Pyelonephritis is an acute and severe form of UTI that specifically affects the kidneys. It occurs when bacteria, commonly Escherichia coli (E. coli), ascend from the lower urinary tract, such as the bladder or ureters, into the kidneys. This ascent can occur due to untreated or inadequately treated UTIs, allowing bacteria to reach and infect the kidneys.

*Pathophysiology of Pyelonephritis:*

Bacteria that reach the kidneys trigger an intense inflammatory response within the renal tissue. This inflammatory reaction causes kidney tissue damage, resulting in symptoms such as severe back pain, high fever, chills, nausea, and vomiting. The infection can affect one or both kidneys.

*Risk Factors and Progression:*

Untreated or recurrent UTIs significantly heighten the risk of developing pyelonephritis. The progression from a standard UTI to pyelonephritis underscores the importance of timely diagnosis and treatment to prevent bacteria from reaching and infecting the kidneys.

## Complications and Scarring

*Kidney Damage and Scarring:*

Severe or recurrent pyelonephritis can cause substantial kidney damage. Prolonged inflammation and untreated infections can lead to the formation of scar tissue within the kidneys, affecting their structure and function.

*Impairment of Renal Function:*

Kidney damage due to pyelonephritis may impair renal function, leading to decreased filtration capabilities and compromising the kidneys' ability to regulate fluids, electrolytes, and waste products in the body.

*Chronic Kidney Issues:*

Prolonged or recurrent kidney infections, particularly if left untreated, may contribute to chronic kidney issues, such as chronic kidney disease (CKD). CKD involves a gradual loss of kidney function over time and can eventually progress to kidney failure if not managed appropriately.

*Clinical Management and Prevention*:

Prompt diagnosis and effective treatment of pyelonephritis are crucial to prevent kidney damage and complications. Management involves appropriate antibiotic therapy to eliminate the infection and alleviate symptoms. Patients may require close monitoring, especially those prone to recurrent infections, to prevent further complications and preserve renal function.

## UTIs and Other Urinary Tract Disorders

*Interstitial Cystitis (IC)*

*Understanding Interstitial Cystitis (IC):*

Interstitial cystitis is a chronic and challenging bladder condition characterized by pelvic pain, urgency, frequency of urination, and sometimes discomfort during sexual intercourse. Unlike typical UTIs, IC isn't primarily caused by bacterial infections but rather involves complex changes in the bladder lining and nerve signaling.

*Potential Connection with UTIs:*

While the exact cause of IC remains unclear, recurrent UTIs or bladder infections may contribute to the development or worsening of IC symptoms in some individuals. Frequent inflammation or damage to the bladder from recurrent UTIs might trigger or exacerbate IC symptoms in susceptible individuals.

*Inflammation and IC Onset:*

It's hypothesized that chronic inflammation or recurring insults to the bladder, such as those seen in recurrent UTIs, may lead to alterations in the bladder lining or nerve signaling, contributing to the development of IC in some cases.

## Urethritis and UTIs

*Understanding Urethritis:*

Urethritis refers to inflammation of the urethra, often caused by bacterial infections (like those causing UTIs), sexually transmitted infections (STIs), or other non-infectious factors. The common symptom of urethritis is discomfort or pain during urination.

*Relation to UTIs:*

UTIs and urethritis can coexist or have overlapping symptoms due to similar underlying causes. UTIs, particularly those affecting the lower urinary tract, can potentially spread to the urethra, causing inflammation and leading to urethritis. Additionally, predisposing factors like improper hygiene or sexual activity can contribute to both conditions.

*Differentiation and Diagnostic Challenges:*

Distinguishing between UTIs and urethritis can pose diagnostic challenges due to similar symptoms. However, urethritis may persist or recur independently of UTIs, requiring different treatment approaches.

## Understanding Recurrent UTIs and Related Disorders
**Contributing Factors to Recurrent UTIs**

*Anatomical Abnormalities:*

Structural variations in the urinary tract, such as anatomical abnormalities like urinary tract obstructions, kidney stones, or vesicoureteral reflux (VUR), can predispose individuals to recurrent UTIs. These abnormalities can create pockets where bacteria thrive or disrupt the normal flow of urine, increasing the risk of infections.

*Immune System Deficiencies:*

Weakened immune defenses due to conditions like HIV/AIDS, diabetes, or immunosuppressive therapies can compromise the body's ability to fight off infections. Individuals with weakened immune systems are more susceptible to recurrent UTIs as their defenses against pathogens are compromised.

*Chronic Health Conditions:*

Chronic health issues like diabetes mellitus, kidney diseases, or neurological conditions affecting bladder function can contribute to recurrent UTIs. Diabetes, for instance, can alter the urinary environment, making it more conducive to bacterial growth.

## Long-Term Implications and Management

*Impact on Quality of Life:*

Recurrent UTIs can significantly impact an individual's quality of life due to the discomfort, pain, and disruption they cause. Frequent medical appointments, antibiotic use, and time spent managing UTIs can affect daily activities and emotional well-being.

*Potential Complications:*

Long-term implications of recurrent UTIs include complications such as kidney damage, chronic kidney disease, sepsis (systemic infection), and an increased risk of antibiotic resistance due to frequent antibiotic use.

*Targeted Management Strategies:*

Management of recurrent UTIs involves multifaceted approaches. Prophylactic antibiotic use might be recommended in specific cases to prevent infections.

Lifestyle modifications, such as adequate hydration, proper hygiene practices, avoiding irritants, and cranberry supplements, can help reduce the risk of recurrences.

*Preventive Measures:*

Preventive measures focus on identifying and addressing underlying causes to prevent future infections. For example, surgical correction of anatomical abnormalities or controlling underlying health conditions to strengthen the immune system can be crucial.

Understanding the complex interplay between recurrent UTIs and related disorders involves identifying predisposing factors, recognizing the potential long-term implications, and implementing targeted management strategies. By addressing underlying factors, adopting preventive measures, and tailoring management approaches, healthcare providers can significantly mitigate the impact of recurrent UTIs on patients' health and well-being.

## Management Strategies for Concurrent Disorders

Managing urinary tract infections (UTIs) alongside other urinary tract disorders requires a comprehensive approach that considers the specific needs and complexities of each condition. Here is an elaboration on the management strategies for concurrent disorders:

## Comprehensive Evaluation

*Thorough Medical Assessment:*

Conducting a comprehensive medical evaluation is crucial to identify and understand the concurrent urinary tract disorders. This evaluation involves a detailed medical history, physical examination, and possibly imaging studies or specialized tests to ascertain the nature and severity of each disorder.

## Tailored Treatment Plans

*Individualized Approaches:*

Designing individualized treatment plans considering the specific nature of each concurrent disorder is essential. This may involve a multidisciplinary team, including urologists, nephrologists, infectious disease specialists, and other healthcare professionals, depending on the disorders involved.

## Specific Management Strategies

*Addressing UTIs:*

For UTIs, prompt diagnosis and targeted antibiotic therapy are vital to eradicate the infection. Antibiotic selection should consider the causative organism's susceptibility, the patient's medical history, and any allergies.

*Treating Other Urinary Tract Disorders:*

Depending on the specific concurrent disorders (such as interstitial cystitis, pyelonephritis, or urethritis), treatment approaches may include a combination of medications, lifestyle modifications, physical therapy, or minimally invasive procedures to alleviate symptoms and manage the underlying condition.

## Holistic Management:

*Lifestyle Modifications:*

Encouraging lifestyle changes that promote urinary tract health is crucial. This may involve increasing fluid intake, maintaining proper hygiene practices, avoiding irritants or triggers, and adopting a balanced diet to support overall urinary health.

*Preventive Measures:*

Implementing preventive measures to minimize the risk of recurrent UTIs or exacerbation of other urinary tract disorders is essential. This may include prophylactic antibiotics, cranberry supplements, or other therapies depending on the individual's needs and condition.

## Ongoing Monitoring and Follow-up

*Regular Follow-ups:*

Monitoring patients with concurrent urinary tract disorders requires regular follow-ups to assess treatment effectiveness, manage complications, and modify treatment plans as needed.

## Patient Education and Support

*Patient Empowerment:*

Educating patients about their conditions, treatment options, and preventive measures is crucial for their active involvement in managing their health. Empowering patients with knowledge helps them make informed decisions and adhere to treatment plans effectively.

# Chapter 7

## Antibiotics for UTI Treatment:

### What Are My Options?

The most commonly prescribed antibiotics for treating urinary tract infections (UTIs) include several medications that have shown efficacy against bacterial infections commonly associated with UTIs. Here's an elaboration on some of these antibiotics:

### Nitrofurantoin (Macrobid)

*Mechanism and Usage:*

Nitrofurantoin is a bactericidal antibiotic that works by interfering with bacterial enzymes involved in the production of bacterial DNA, RNA, and cell wall synthesis. It is effective against a broad spectrum of bacteria commonly responsible for causing UTIs.

Often prescribed for uncomplicated UTIs, Nitrofurantoin is particularly useful against Escherichia coli (E. coli) and other common pathogens. It is generally taken orally as a capsule or tablet form, twice a day for a duration of five to seven days.

*Considerations:*

This antibiotic is well-absorbed orally and primarily excreted through the kidneys, making it a suitable option for treating lower urinary tract infections.

**Trimethoprim/Sulfamethoxazole (Bactrim)**
*Mechanism and Usage:*

Trimethoprim/sulfamethoxazole is a combination antibiotic that works by inhibiting bacterial enzymes involved in the synthesis of folic acid, a critical component for bacterial growth. It exhibits effectiveness against various bacteria causing UTIs.

Often used to treat uncomplicated UTIs, this combination is particularly active against E. coli and some other gram-negative bacteria. The usual regimen involves twice-daily oral doses for approximately three days.

*Considerations:*

The combination of trimethoprim/sulfamethoxazole is well-tolerated, but some individuals may experience allergic reactions or adverse effects, such as gastrointestinal disturbances or skin rashes.


**Fosfomycin (Monurol)**
*Mechanism and Usage:*

Fosfomycin is an antibiotic that inhibits bacterial cell wall synthesis by targeting a specific enzyme essential for bacterial growth. It is known for its effectiveness against a range of bacteria, including E. coli.

Typically prescribed as a single-dose oral sachet, Fosfomycin is a convenient option for treating uncomplicated UTIs.

*Considerations:*

Fosfomycin's single-dose regimen provides an advantage in terms of adherence to treatment, convenience, and efficacy in certain uncomplicated UTI cases.


## Cephalexin (Keflex)
*Mechanism and Usage:*

Cephalexin belongs to the class of antibiotics known as cephalosporins. It works by interfering with the bacteria's cell wall formation, leading to their eventual death. This antibiotic demonstrates effectiveness against a wide range of bacteria commonly associated with complicated UTIs.

Typically prescribed for more severe or complicated UTIs, Cephalexin is often taken orally and is absorbed well from the gastrointestinal tract. The usual dosage regimen involves taking it four times a day, generally for a duration of seven to fourteen days.

*Considerations:*

Cephalexin is a well-tolerated antibiotic but may cause some side effects such as gastrointestinal disturbances, allergic reactions, or, less commonly, mild skin rashes.

### Ciprofloxacin (Cipro)

*Mechanism and Usage:*

Ciprofloxacin is a broad-spectrum fluoroquinolone antibiotic that inhibits bacterial DNA gyrase and topoisomerase, disrupting DNA replication and leading to bacterial cell death. It exhibits effectiveness against a wide array of bacteria causing complicated UTIs.

Often prescribed for complicated or more severe UTIs, Ciprofloxacin is taken orally and is well-absorbed from the gastrointestinal tract. The typical dosage regimen involves taking it twice a day, usually for a duration of seven to fourteen days.

*Considerations:*

Ciprofloxacin is generally well-tolerated, but some individuals may experience side effects such as gastrointestinal upset, dizziness, or tendon inflammation or rupture, especially with prolonged use or in certain patient populations.

It is important to note that the choice of antibiotic may vary depending on the patient's medical history, age, and other factors. Patients should always consult their healthcare provider before taking any antibiotics.

## Antibiotics and Side Effects

*Potential Side Effects:*

Antibiotics are effective in treating UTIs by eliminating bacterial infections. However, they can lead to side effects in some individuals. Common side effects may include gastrointestinal disturbances like nausea, vomiting, or diarrhea. Additionally, allergic reactions, ranging from mild rashes to severe anaphylaxis, may occur in certain cases.

*Importance of Reporting Side Effects:*

Patients taking antibiotics should be vigilant about any adverse reactions. It's crucial to inform their healthcare provider promptly if they experience any side effects while on antibiotic treatment. Timely reporting allows healthcare professionals to assess and manage side effects appropriately, potentially adjusting the treatment plan or providing supportive care.

## Non-Antibiotic Treatments for UTIs

*Hydration and Frequent Urination:*

Drinking plenty of water and urinating frequently help flush out bacteria from the urinary tract, potentially aiding in preventing or alleviating UTIs. Adequate hydration maintains urine flow and dilutes bacteria, reducing the risk of infection.

*Over-the-Counter Pain Relievers:*

Over-the-counter pain relievers like ibuprofen or acetaminophen can help manage discomfort or pain associated with UTI symptoms, such as urinary urgency, frequency, or mild discomfort.

*Cranberry Juice:*

Some studies suggest that cranberry juice may have properties that prevent bacteria from adhering to the urinary tract lining, potentially reducing the risk of UTIs. However, the evidence is not conclusive, and more research is needed to establish its efficacy definitively.

## Considerations and Recommendations:

*Patient Education:*

Patients should be educated about the importance of staying hydrated, maintaining good urinary habits, and managing mild symptoms with over-the-counter pain relievers if needed.

*Consultation with Healthcare Provider:*

While non-antibiotic treatments like increased hydration or cranberry juice may aid in preventing or managing UTIs, patients should consult their healthcare provider before starting any new treatment regimen. Healthcare professionals can provide guidance tailored to individual needs, considering the severity and recurrence of UTIs, medical history, and possible interactions with existing medications.

Antibiotics are effective in treating UTIs, but they may cause side effects, which patients should report to their healthcare provider promptly. Non-antibiotic treatments, including adequate hydration, frequent urination, over-the-counter pain relievers, and potential remedies like cranberry juice, may complement antibiotic therapy or be used as preventive measures. However, it's crucial for patients to consult with healthcare providers before starting any alternative treatments and to follow their recommendations for UTI management.

## Novel Strategies in Combating UTIs
### NRF2 Pathway's Role in UTI Management:

The research conducted by Baylor College of Medicine and Washington University School of Medicine has unveiled a promising avenue in combating urinary tract infections (UTIs). The study elucidates a delicate interplay within the body during UTIs—balancing the immune response against the invading bacteria while minimizing potential tissue damage. The NRF2 pathway emerged as a pivotal regulator in maintaining this equilibrium. By modulating this pathway, specifically with dimethyl fumarate (DMF), an FDA-approved anti-inflammatory drug known to activate NRF2, researchers observed a remarkable reduction in both tissue damage and bacterial burden in animal models of UTI. This discovery opens doors to potential future treatments harnessing NRF2 activation to manage UTIs more effectively.

## Electrofulguration as a Promising Minimally Invasive Procedure:

In another study, electrofulguration, a minimally invasive procedure targeting inflamed and infected bladder tissue, has shown promise in providing relief for individuals dealing with recurrent UTIs. This technique involves precisely zapping and eliminating inflamed tissue within the bladder. This innovative approach presents a potential alternative or complementary strategy to conventional treatments for individuals suffering from frequent UTIs, offering hope for those seeking non-pharmacological interventions.

## Non-Prescription Steps in UTI Management:

While antibiotics remain the cornerstone of UTI treatment, studies underscore the potential for non-prescription approaches in managing milder cases. Research suggests that up to 40% of bladder infections can be resolved through non-prescription measures. Increasing water intake helps flush out bacteria from the urinary tract. Pain relief medications, such as ibuprofen, can alleviate discomfort associated with UTIs. This highlights the significance of adopting simple yet effective self-care practices that may aid in alleviating symptoms and potentially clearing milder UTIs without the necessity of antibiotics.

These emerging research findings illuminate a landscape of hope in UTI management, showcasing innovative strategies beyond conventional antibiotic treatments. The NRF2 pathway modulation with DMF and electrofulguration offer promising avenues for future therapies, while the acknowledgment of non-prescription steps underscores the potential for holistic approaches in mitigating milder UTIs. While antibiotics remain crucial, these studies advocate for a comprehensive approach, embracing both pharmacological and non-pharmacological options, thus broadening the horizon for UTI management.

# Conclusion

In concluding this comprehensive book on bladder health, our journey has been one of understanding, empowerment, and proactive care. Throughout these pages, we've ventured into the intricate world of urinary tract infections (UTIs), delving into their causes, symptoms, treatments, preventive measures, and alternative therapies. Our goal has been to equip readers with a holistic understanding of bladder health, empowering them to take charge of their well-being.

Bladder health is a crucial yet often overlooked aspect of overall wellness. By unraveling the complexities of UTIs, we've strived to provide a roadmap for readers to navigate this terrain with confidence and knowledge. From understanding the anatomical nuances of the urinary tract to recognizing the vulnerabilities that predispose individuals to infections, we've aimed to shed light on the intricacies of bladder health.

The power of prevention has been a recurring theme throughout this book. We've emphasized the significance of hygiene practices, hydration, and lifestyle choices in mitigating the risk of UTIs. By fostering an awareness of symptoms and encouraging prompt medical attention, we've aimed to instill a proactive mindset—one that values early detection and intervention.

However, this book is not merely a compendium of facts; it's a call to action. It's an invitation to embark on a journey of continuous learning and application. Bladder health is a dynamic realm, and staying informed about the latest research, innovations, and advancements is pivotal in nurturing one's well-being.

The essence of this book lies not just in the knowledge shared, but in the application of this knowledge in daily life. It's about adopting healthier habits, engaging in open dialogues with healthcare providers, and making informed decisions that prioritize bladder health.

I encourage each reader to embrace the principles of proactive bladder health. This journey is one of empowerment—an opportunity to seize control, make informed choices, and lead a life characterized by vitality and wellness. By applying the insights garnered from this book, may each step taken be a stride toward a healthier, more fulfilling life.

As we draw this journey to a close, let us remember that proactive bladder health is not a destination but a continuous pursuit—one that thrives on knowledge, action, and a steadfast commitment to personal well-being. Here's to empowered choices, proactive care, and a future abundant in vibrant health and vitality.